Keto Diet: Breakfast Recipes

Top 50 Tasty Recipes of 2021

SUMMARY

INTRODUZIONE

Breakfast is always the most important meal of the day, from here you collect all the energy you need to face the day in the best way!

I wrote this book thinking of you, who care about your figure, your physical fitness and want to have breakfast with a super good and protein meal.

Ketosis is very important and here you will find all the recipes and ingredients needed to develop it in the best way.

So Good morning to all of you, let's start the day in the best way together.

BREAKFAST AND SMOOTHIE RECIPES

EGG AND SAUSAGE CASSEROLE

Ingredients

- 1 lb of ground breakfast sausage

- ½ cup chopped onion

- ½ chopped green pepper

- 2 chopped mushrooms

- 12 large eggs

- 1 cup almond milk

- 1 tsp. salt

- ½ tsp. pepper

- ¼ tsp. thyme

- ¼ tsp. rosemary

- tomatoes/salsa for garnish, if desired

Instructions

1. Preheat oven to 350° F. Grease a 9×13 pan.

2. Cook breakfast sausage in a pan. When the sausage is cooked, add the chopped onion, green pepper and mushrooms and cook for a few min

3. Combine the eggs, almond milk, salt, pepper, thyme and rosemary in a large bowl. Beat well. Add the vegetables and the meat mixture and mix to combine. Pour into baking pan and bake for 30 min (or until the inserted knife comes out clean).

4. Serve with tomatoes or salsa, if desired.

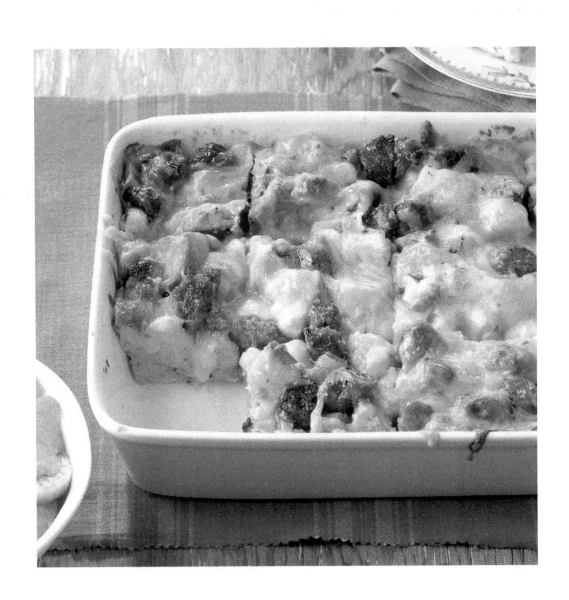

CAPRESE OMELET

Ingredients

- 2 Tbsp butter

- 2 to 4 eggs

- salt and pepper garlic powder (optional)

- 1 small tomato, diced

- 3-4 fresh basil leaves, finely chopped

- ¼ cup grated mozzarella

- optional olive oil

Instructions

1. Melt butter in a medium-sized skillet over medium heat.

2. Place eggs in the pan and sprinkle half the tomatoes, basil and cheese on top.

3. Cook until ready, turning if necessary.

4. Remove and cover quickly with the other half of the tomatoes, basil and cheese and sprinkle with olive oil if desired.

Prep time:5 min; **Servings:** 2

Macros: Cal 366 Carbs 4.5 g Protein 14.1 g Fat 33.2 g Saturated Fat 18.1 g Cholesterol 392 mg Sodium 489 mg Fiber 1.1 g Sugar 3.1 g

CREAMY KALE BAKED EGGS

Ingredients

- 2 large eggs

- Coconut Milk

- Creamed kale

- 2 Tbsp Roasted Red Peppers

- Cherry Tomatoes

- ½ cup Grated Mozzarella Cheese (optional)

Instructions

1. Preheat the oven to 400° F.

2. Grease 4 small baking pans.

3. Roasted red peppers at the end of cooking.

4. Divide creamed kale into 4 separate piles.

5. Cover each with chopped tomatoes and cheese.

6. Use a spoon to create a small notch in each pile and fill with an egg.

7. Bake for 15-20 min

Prep time:25 min; **Servings:** 4

Macros: Cal 388 Fat 34.9g Saturated Fat 20.4g Carbs 6g Fiber 0.5g Sugar 0.5g Protein 14

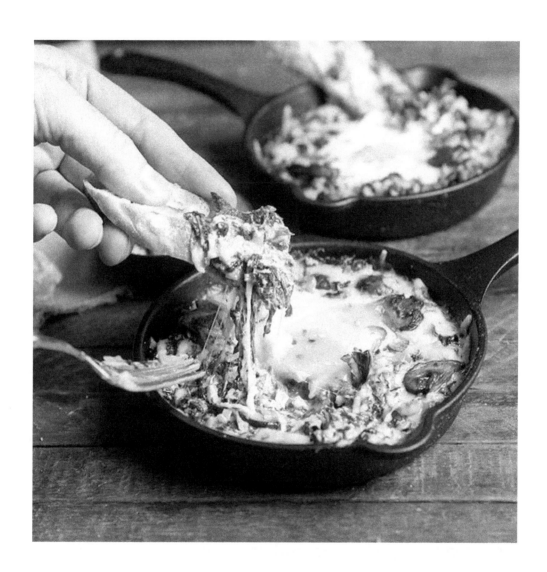

EASY ASPARAGUS QUICHE

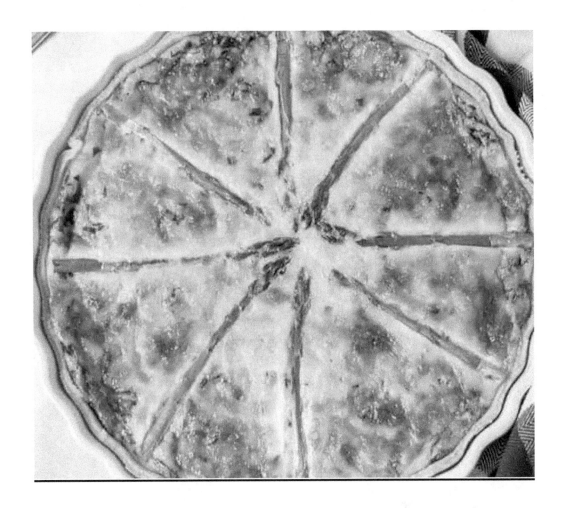

Ingredients:

- 10 eggs

- 2 lbs. asparagus, trimmed and remove ends

- 3 tbsp. olive oil

- Pepper

- Salt

Instructions:

1. Preheat the oven to 425 F.

2. Arrange asparagus on the baking sheet. Drizzle 1 tablespoon olive oil over asparagus.

3. Roast asparagus in preheated oven for 15 minutes.

4. In a mixing bowl, whisk eggs with remaining oil, pepper, and salt.

5. Transfer roasted asparagus in a quiche pan. Pour egg mixture over asparagus.

6. Bake at 350 F for 30 minutes or until egg sets.

7. Slice and serve.

Prep time: 10 minutes **Servings:** 8

Cooking Time: 45 minutes

Nutrition: Calories 146 Fat 10.9 g Carbohydrates 4.8 g Sugar 2.6 g Protein 9.4 g Cholesterol 205 mg

BAKED BREAKFAST FRITTATA

Ingredients:

- 12 eggs

- 1 tsp garlic powder

- 2 1/2 cups mushrooms, chopped

- 1 cup cheddar cheese, shredded

- 1 red bell pepper, chopped

- 1 small onion, chopped

- 1 cup ham, chopped

- 1 1/2 cups asparagus, chopped

- Pepper

- Salt

Instructions

- Preheat the oven to 375 F. Grease 9*13-inch baking pan.

- Add asparagus, mushrooms, cheese, bell pepper, onion, and ham into the prepared pan.

- In a bowl, whisk eggs with garlic powder, pepper, and salt.

- Pour egg mixture over vegetables and stir gently.

- Bake for 25-35 minutes or until frittata is set.

- Slice and serve.

Preparation Time: 10 minutes **; Servings:** 12

Cooking Time: 35 minutes

Nutrition: Calories 132 Fat 8.6 g Carbohydrates 3.5 g Sugar 1.8 g Protein 10.8 g Cholesterol 180 mg

CAULIFLOWER BREAKFAST CASSEROLE

Ingredients:

- 10 eggs

- 4 cups cauliflower rice

- 12 oz. bacon, cooked and crumbled

- 1/2 cup heavy whipping cream

- 1 tsp paprika

- 8 oz. cheddar cheese, shredded

- 1/4 tsp pepper

- 1 tsp salt

Instructions

1. Preheat the oven to 350 F. Grease 2-quart casserole dish.

2. Spread cauliflower rice into the prepared dish and top with half cheddar cheese.

3. In a bowl, whisk eggs with cream, paprika, pepper, and salt and pour over cauliflower. Top with remaining cheese and bacon.

4. Bake for 45 minutes.

5. Serve and enjoy.

Preparation Time: 10 minutes; **Servings:** 6

Cooking Time: 45 minutes

Nutrition: Calories 637 Fat 48.5 g Carbohydrates 6.9 g Sugar 3.5 g Protein 42.5 g Cholesterol 389 mg

TURKEY CHEESE FRITTATA

Ingredients:

- 8 eggs

- 8 oz. turkey deli meat

- 2 tbsp. cheddar cheese, shredded

- 2 tbsp. parmesan cheese, shredded

- 1/2 tsp oregano

- 1/2 tsp thyme

- 1/4 tsp pepper

- 1/4 tsp salt

Instructions

1. Preheat the oven to 350 F.

2. Line an 8-inch skillet with the turkey deli meat.

3. In a bowl, whisk eggs with oregano, thyme, pepper, and salt. Pour egg mixture over meat.

4. Sprinkle parmesan cheese and cheddar cheese on top.

5. Bake for 20-25 minutes.

6. Serve and enjoy.

Preparation Time: 10 minutes; **Servings:** 8

Cooking Time: 25 minutes

Nutrition: Calories 108 Fat 6 g Carbohydrates 1.2 g Sugar 0.4 g Protein 11.8 g Cholesterol 178 mg

EASY CHEESE QUICHE

Ingredients:

- 12 eggs

- 12 tbsp. butter, melted

- 4 oz. cream cheese, softened

- 8 oz. cheddar cheese, grated

- Pepper

- Salt

Instructions

1. Spread cheddar cheese into the 9-5-inch pie pan.

2. Add eggs, cream cheese, butter, pepper, and salt into the blender and blend until well combined.

3. Pour egg mixture over cheese in pie pan and bake at 325 F for 45 minutes.

4. Slice and serve.

Preparation Time: 10 minutes; **Servings:** 6

Cooking Time: 45 minutes

Nutrition: Calories 548 Fat 50.9 g Carbohydrates 1.7 g Sugar 0.9 g Protein 22.2 g Cholesterol 449 mg

ZUCCHINI BACON BAKE

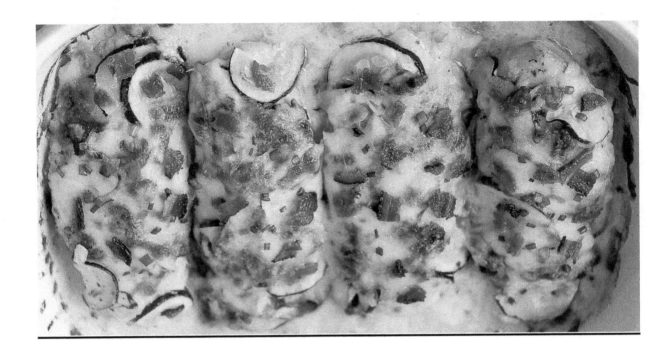

Ingredients:

- 8 egg whites

- 3 tbsp. bacon, crumbled

- 1/4 cup unsweetened almond milk

- 3 wedges Swiss cheese

- 1/2 cup cottage cheese

- 2 cups shredded zucchini

- 1/2 tsp salt

Instructions

1. Preheat the oven to 350 F. Grease 8*8-inch casserole dish.

2. Add shredded zucchini into the prepared dish.

3. Add egg, bacon, milk, Swiss cheese, cottage cheese, and salt into the blender and blend until smooth.

4. Pour blended egg mixture over shredded zucchini.

5. Bake in preheated oven for 30 minutes.

6. Serve and enjoy.

Preparation Time: 10 minutes ; **Servings:** 8

Cooking Time: 30 minutes

Nutrition: Calories 114 Fat 6.4 g Carbohydrates 2.4 g Sugar 0.9 g Protein 11.4 g Cholesterol 19 mg

JALAPENO BREAKFAST CASSEROLE

Ingredients:

- 12 eggs

- 2 jalapeno peppers, sliced

- 4 oz. cream cheese, cut into cubes

- 1 cup cheddar cheese, shredded

- 1/2 cup bacon, cooked and chopped

- 1 cup heavy whipping cream

- 1/2 tsp pepper

- 1/4 tsp salt

Instructions

1. Preheat the oven to 350 F. Grease 9*13-inch baking pan and set aside.

2. In a large bowl, whisk eggs with cream cheese, cream, pepper, and salt and pour into the prepared pan.

3. Sprinkle jalapeno slices, bacon, and 3/4 cup cheddar cheese evenly over egg mixture.

4. Bake for 25-30 minutes. Remove pan from oven and top with remaining cheese and bake for 5 minutes more.

5. Serve and enjoy.

Preparation Time: 10 minutes; **Servings:** 10

Cooking Time: 30 minutes

Nutrition: Calories 209 Fat 17.8 g Carbohydrates 1.5 g Sugar 0.6 g Protein 11 g Cholesterol 238 mg

RANCH BREAKFAST QUICHE

Ingredients:

- 8 eggs

- 1 cup sour cream

- 1 tbsp. ranch seasoning

- 1 1/2 cups cheddar cheese, shredded

- 1 lb. ground Italian sausage

Instructions

1. Preheat the oven to 350 F.

2. Brown the sausage in an oven-safe skillet and drain well.

3. In a bowl, whisk eggs with ranch seasoning, and sour cream. Stir in cheddar cheese.

4. Pour egg mixture over sausage in skillet. Cover skillet with foil.

5. Bake for 30 minutes. Remove foil and bake for 25 minutes more.

6. Serve and enjoy.

Preparation Time: 10 minutes; **Servings:** 6

Cooking Time: 55 minutes

Nutrition: Calories 511 Fat 40.6 g Carbohydrates 3.8 g Sugar 2 g Protein 29 g Cholesterol 318 mg

BROCCOLI EGG BAKE

Ingredients:

- 12 eggs

- 2 cups broccoli florets, chopped

- 1/2 cup cheddar cheese, shredded

- 3/4 tsp onion powder

- 1/2 cup unsweetened coconut milk

- Pepper

- Salt

Instructions

- Preheat the oven to 350 F. Grease 9*13-inch baking dish.

- In a bowl, whisk eggs with cheese, onion powder, milk, pepper, and salt. Stir in broccoli.

- Pour egg mixture into the prepared dish and bake for 30 minutes.

- Slice and serve.

Preparation Time: 10 minutes; **Servings:** 6

Cooking Time: 30 minutes

Nutrition: Calories 221 Fat 16.7 g Carbohydrates 4.2 g Sugar 2 g Protein 14.8 g Cholesterol 337 mg

SAUSAGE RICOTTA CHEESE CASSEROLE

Ingredients:

- 10 eggs

- 2 1/2 lbs. Italian sausage

- 1 tbsp. fresh basil, chopped

- 12 cherry tomatoes, halved

- 16 oz. ricotta cheese, cut into cubes

- 4 oz. cream cheese

- 1 tsp salt

Instructions

- Preheat the oven to 400 F.

- Add sausage into the casserole dish and bake for 20 minutes. Once done, drain sausage well and break in small pieces using a masher.

- In a bowl, whisk eggs with cream cheese until smooth and pour over sausage. Season with salt. Sprinkle ricotta cheese cubes, tomatoes, and basil on top.

- Bake for 35-40 minutes more.

- Serve and enjoy.

Preparation Time: 10 minutes; **Servings:** 12

Cooking Time: 55 minutes

Nutrition: Calories 480 Fat 37 g Carbohydrates 7.3 g Sugar 3.7 g Protein 29.1 g Cholesterol 238 mg

EASY CHEESE EGG BAKE

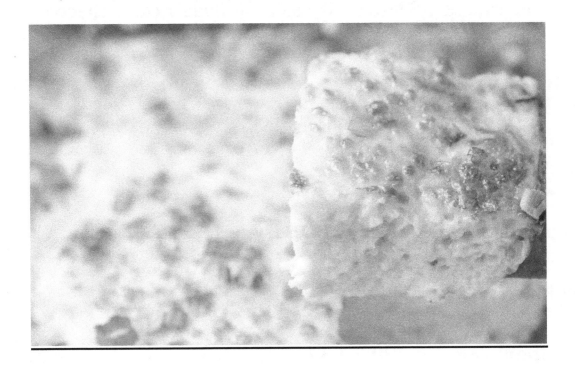

Ingredients:

- 4 eggs

- 1/3 cup half and half

- 4 oz. cream cheese

- Pinch of salt

Instructions

1. Preheat the oven to 350 F.

2. Add eggs, half and half, cream cheese, and salt into the blender and blend until smooth.

3. Pour egg mixture into the greased baking dish and bake for 30 minutes.

4. Serve and enjoy.

Preparation Time: 10 minutes; **Servings:** 4

Cooking Time: 30 minutes

Nutrition: Calories 188 Fat 16.6 g Carbohydrates 2 g Sugar 0.4 g Protein 8.3 g Cholesterol 202 mg

ZUCCHINI EGG CASSEROLE

Ingredients:

- 10 eggs

- 3 cherry tomatoes, halved

- 1/2 cup mushrooms, sliced

- 1/3 cup ham, chopped

- 1 small zucchini, sliced into rounds

- 1/2 cup spinach

- 2/3 cup heavy cream

- Pepper

- Salt

Instructions

1. Preheat the oven to 350 F. Grease 9*13-inch pan and set aside.

2. In a large bowl, whisk eggs with heavy cream, pepper, and salt. Stir in tomatoes, mushrooms, ham, zucchini, and spinach.

3. Pour egg mixture in prepared pan and bake for 30-35 minutes.

4. Serve and enjoy.

Preparation Time: 10 minutes; **Servings:** 8

Cooking Time: 30 minutes

Nutrition: Calories 134 Fat 9.8 g Carbohydrates 3.4 g Sugar 2 g Protein 8.8 g Cholesterol 222 mg

SAUSAGE EGG OMELET

Ingredients:

- 7 eggs

- 1 tsp mustard

- 2 cups cheddar cheese, shredded

- 3/4 cup heavy whipping cream

- 1/4 onion, chopped

- 1/2 green bell pepper, chopped

- 1 lb. breakfast sausage

- 1/4 tsp pepper

- 1/2 tsp salt

Instructions

1. Preheat the oven to 350 F. Grease 9*13-inch casserole dish and set aside.

2. Brown the sausage in a pan. Add onion and bell pepper and cook until onion is softened. Remove pan from heat.

3. In a bowl, whisk eggs with mustard, 1 3/4 cups of cheese, cream, pepper, and salt.

4. Spread sausage mixture into the prepared casserole. Pour egg mixture on top of the sausage mixture and top with remaining cheese.

5. Bake for 20-23 minutes.

6. Serve and enjoy.

Preparation Time: 10 minutes; **Servings:** 12

Cooking Time: 23 minutes

Nutrition: Calories 271 Fat 22.4 g Carbohydrates 1.4 g Sugar 0.7 g Protein 15.6 g Cholesterol 157 mg

SAUSAGE BREAKFAST CASSEROLE

Ingredients:

- 12 eggs

- 1 tbsp. hot sauce

- 3/4 cup heavy whipping cream

- 2 cups cheddar cheese, shredded

- 12 oz. breakfast sausage

- Pepper

- Salt

Instructions

1. Preheat the oven to 350 F. Grease 9*13-inch casserole dish.

2. Heat a large pan over medium-high heat.

3. Add sausage to the pan and break with a wooden spoon and cook for 5-7 minutes or until meat is no longer pink.

4. Transfer cooked sausage into the prepared dish and spread evenly.

5. In a large bowl, whisk eggs with hot sauce, cream, cheese, pepper, and salt.

6. Pour egg mixture over sausage and bake for 30-40 minutes.

7. Serve and enjoy.

Preparation Time: 10 minutes; **Servings:** 8

Cooking Time: 40 minutes

Nutrition: Calories 391 Fat 32.2 g Carbohydrates 1.2 g Sugar 0.7 g Protein 23.8 g Cholesterol 326 mg

CHICKEN CHEESE QUICHE

Ingredients:

- 8 eggs

- 1/2 tsp oregano

- 1/4 tsp onion powder

- 1/4 tsp garlic powder

- 1/4 cup mozzarella cheese, shredded

- 5 oz. cooked chicken breast, chopped

- 1/4 tsp pepper

- 1/2 tsp salt

Instructions

1. Preheat the oven to 350 F.

2. In a bowl, whisk eggs with oregano, onion powder, pepper, and salt. Stir in cheese and chicken.

3. Pour egg mixture in pie pan and bake for 35-45 minutes.

4. Slice and serve.

Preparation Time: 10 minutes ; **Servings:** 4

Cooking Time: 45 minutes

Nutrition: Calories 173 Fat 10 g Carbohydrates 1.2 g Sugar 0.8 g Protein 19.2 g Cholesterol 351 mg

EGG & BACON CUPS

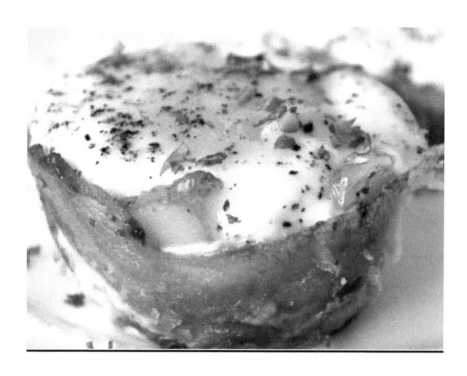

Ingredients:

- 2 bacon strips

- 2 large eggs

- Handful of fresh spinach

- ¼ cup cheese

- Salt and pepper to taste

Instructions

- Preheat your oven to 400 degrees Fahrenheit.

- Fry bacon in a skillet over medium heat, drain the oil and keep them on the side.

- Take muffin tin and grease with oil.

- Line with a slice of bacon, press down the bacon well, making sure that the ends are sticking out (to be used as handles).

- Take a bowl and beat eggs.

- Drain and pat the spinach dry.

- Add the spinach to the eggs.

- Add a quarter of the mixture in each of your muffin tins.

- Sprinkle cheese and season.

- Bake for 15 minutes.

- Enjoy!

Preparation Time: 10 minutes **Servings:** 6

Cooking Time: 15 minutes

Nutrition: Calories: 101 Fat: 7 g Carbohydrates: 2 g Protein: 8 g Fiber: 1 g Net Carbs: 1 g

MOZZARELLA STICKS WITH BACON

Ingredients:

- 4 bacon strips

- 2 mozzarella string cheese pieces

- Sunflower oil, as needed

Instructions

- Take a heavy-duty skillet over medium heat and add about 2 inches of oil.

- Heat it to 350 degrees Fahrenheit.

- Have each string cheese to 8 pieces.

- Wrap each piece of string cheese with a strip of bacon and secure it using a toothpick.

- Cook the sticks in oil for 2 minutes until the bacon is browned.

- Place the sticks on a plate lined with a kitchen towel and drain.

- Serve!

Preparation Time: 10 minutes **Servings:** 2

Cooking Time: 5 minutes

Nutrition: Calories: 278 **Fat:** 15g **Net Carbohydrates:** 3g **Protein:** 32g **Fiber:** 1g **Net Carbs:** 2g

CINNAMON COCONUT PORRIDGE

Ingredients:

- 1 cup of water

- 1/2 cup 36% heavy cream

- ½ cup unsweetened dried coconut, shredded

- 1 tablespoon oat bran

- 1 tablespoon flaxseed meal

- 1/2 tablespoon butter

- 1½ teaspoon stevia

- ½ teaspoon cinnamon

- Sea salt, as needed

- Toppings (blueberries or banana slices)

Instructions

1. Add the ingredients mentioned above to a small pot, mix well until fully incorporated.

2. Transfer the pot to your stove over medium-low heat and bring the mix to a slow boil.

3. Stir well and remove the heat.

4. Divide the mixture into equal servings and let them sit for 10 minutes.

5. Top with your desired toppings and enjoy!

Preparation Time: 5 minutes **Servings:** 4

Cooking Time: 5 minutes

Nutrition: Calories: 171 Fat: 16g Net Carbohydrates: 6g Protein: 2g Fiber: 2g Carbohydrates: 8g

MIXED BERRY SMOOTHIE

Ingredients:

- ¼ cup frozen blueberries

- ¼ cup frozen blackberries

- 1 cup unsweetened almond milk

- 1 teaspoon vanilla bean extract

- 3 teaspoon flaxseed

- 1 scoop chilled Greek yogurt

- Stevia, as needed

Instructions

1. Mix everything in a blender and emulsify them.

2. Pulse the mixture four times until you have your desired thickness.

3. The smoothie is ready. Pour and enjoy it!

Preparation Time: 4 minutes **Servings:** 2

Cooking Time: 0 minutes

Nutrition: Calories: 221 Fat: 9g Net Carbohydrates: 8g Protein: 21g Fiber: 2g Carbohydrates: 10g

COCONUT PORRIDGE

Ingredients:

- 2 tablespoons coconut flour

- 2 tablespoons vanilla protein powder

- 3 tablespoons Golden Flaxseed Meal

- 1½ cups almond milk, unsweetened

- Powdered Erythritol

Instructions

1. Take a bowl, mix in flaxseed meal, protein powder, coconut flour, and mix well.

2. Add mix to a saucepan (placed over medium heat).

3. Add almond milk and stir, let the mixture thicken.

4. Add your desired amount of sweetener and serve.

5. Enjoy!

Preparation Time: 15 minutes **Servings:** 2

Cooking Time: 0 minutes

Nutrition: Calories: 259 **Fat:** 13g **Carbohydrates:** 5g **Protein:** 16g
Fiber: 2g **Net Carbohydrates:** 7g

SWISS CHARD OMELET

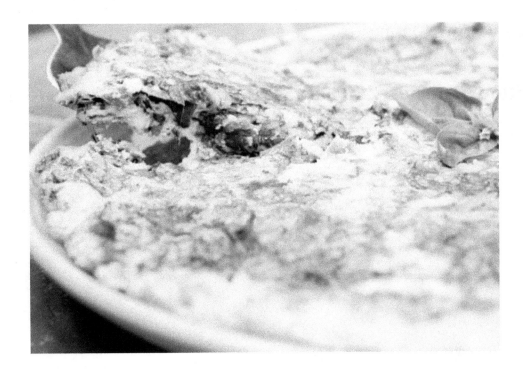

Ingredients:

- 2 eggs, lightly beaten

- 2 cups Swiss chard, sliced

- 1 tablespoon butter

- ½ teaspoon garlic salt

- Fresh pepper

Instructions

1. Take a non-stick frying pan and place it over medium-low heat.

2. Once the butter melts, add Swiss chard and stir cook for 2 minutes.

3. Pour egg into the pan and gently stir them into Swiss chard.

4. Season with garlic salt and pepper.

5. Cook for 2 minutes.

6. Serve and enjoy!

Preparation Time: 5 minutes **Servings:** 2

Cooking Time: 5 minutes

Nutrition: Calories: 260 Fat: 21g Net Carbohydrates: 4g Protein: 14g Fiber: 1g Carbohydrates: 5g

SCRAMBLED PESTO EGGS

Ingredients:

- 2 large whole eggs

- 1/2 tablespoon butter

- 1/2 tablespoon pesto

- 1 tablespoon creamed coconut milk

- Salt, as needed

- pepper, as needed

Instructions

1. Take a bowl and crack open your eggs.

2. Sprinkle with salt and pepper to your taste.

3. Pour eggs into a pan.

4. Add butter and introduce heat.

5. Cook on low heat and gently add pesto.

6. Once the egg is cooked and scrambled, remove heat.

7. Spoon in coconut cream and mix well.

8. Turn on the heat and cook on low for a while until you have a creamy texture.

9. Serve and enjoy!

Preparation Time: 5 minutes **Servings:** 2

Cooking Time: 5 minutes

Nutrition: Calories: 467 Fat: 41g Carbohydrates: 3g Protein: 20g Fiber: 2g Net Carbohydrates: 1g

MUSHROOM FRITTATA

Ingredients:

- 2 tablespoon butter

- 4 whole eggs

- 1-ounce baby spinach, diced

- 1/2 cup fontina cheese, diced

- ½ cup red onion, chopped

- 1/2 cup mushrooms, sliced

- 1/4 cup Greek yogurt, plain

- 1/8 teaspoon nutmeg

Instructions

1. Preheat your oven to 350 degrees Fahrenheit.

2. Take an iron skillet and place it over medium heat.

3. Add butter and let the butter melt.

4. Add onion and mushrooms and cook until translucent.

5. Take a bowl and whip eggs, sour cream, and spinach.

6. Add a ½ cup of cheese.

7. Add butter to the skillet with onion and mushroom and place it over medium.

8. Pour egg mixture and let it cook for 4 minutes (no stir).

9. Remove heat and sprinkle the rest of the cheese.

10. Transfer to oven and bake for 29 minutes.

11. Serve and enjoy!

Preparation Time: 9 minutes **Servings:** 2

Cooking Time: 44 minutes

Nutrition: Calories: 359 Fat: 14g Net Carbohydrates: 14g Protein: 43g Fiber: 2g Carbohydrates: 16g

DEVIL EGGS

Ingredients:

- 4 whole hard-boiled eggs

- 2 tablespoon mayonnaise (Keto friendly or homemade)

- 1 tablespoon spicy brown mustard

- 1 tablespoon green chilies, diced

Instructions

1. Boil your eggs for 9 minutes.

2. Transfer boiled eggs to a water bath and peel the skin.

3. Slice the egg in half and scoop out the yolks.

4. Take a bowl and add yolks, mayonnaise, chilies, and mustard.

5. Mix well and transfer the mixture back to the egg white shells.

6. Enjoy!

Preparation Time: 9 minutes **Servings:** 2

Cooking Time: 11 minutes

Nutrition: Calories: 202 Fat: 15g Net Carbohydrates: 3g Protein: 12g Fiber: 2g Carbohydrates: 5g

SPINACH DIP

Ingredients:

- 5-ounce Spinach, raw

- 1 cup Greek yogurt

- ½ tablespoon onion powder

- ¼ teaspoon garlic salt

- Black pepper, to taste

- ¼ teaspoon Greek Seasoning

Instructions

1. Add the listed ingredients in a blender.

2. Thoroughly emulsify.

3. Season and serve.

Preparation Time: 4 minutes **Servings:** 2

Cooking Time: 0 minutes

Nutrition: Calories: 101 Fat: 4g Net Carbohydrates: 4g Protein: 10g Fiber: 2g Carbohydrates: 6g

COTTAGE CHEESE HOTCAKE

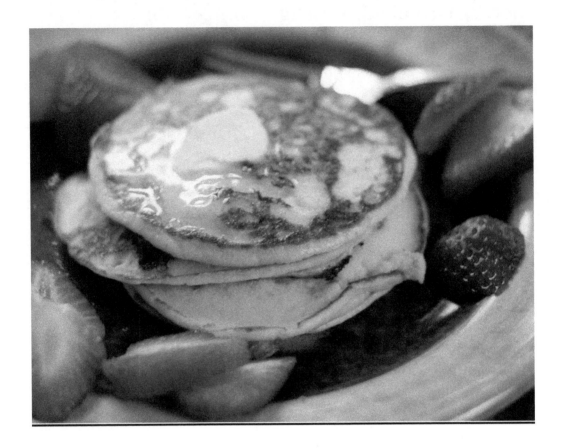

Ingredients:

- 1 cup full–fat cottage cheese

- ½ cup full-fat ricotta cheese

- 2 whole eggs

- ¼ cup coconut cream

- ½ teaspoon baking powder

- 1 teaspoon vanilla extract

- Butter for frying

- 2 teaspoon almond butter

Instructions

1. Add cottage cheese, ricotta cheese, eggs, coconut cream to a bowl, whisk well.

2. Add ground almond, coconut flour, baking powder, vanilla extra, and whisk until smooth.

3. Preheat the non-stick frying pan over medium heat.

4. Add a knob of butter.

5. Once butter melts, add dollops of batter onto a hot pan.

6. Once bubbles appear, flip the pancakes over.

7. Serve with almond butter.

8. Enjoy!

Preparation Time: 10 minutes **Servings:** 2

Cooking Time: 5-10 minutes

Nutrition: Calories: 690 **Fat:** 48g **Carbohydrates:** 16g **Protein: 40g Fiber:** 3g **Net Carbohydrates:** 13g

PEPPERONI OMELET

Ingredients:

- 3 eggs

- 7 pepperoni slices

- 1 teaspoon coconut cream

- Salt

- freshly ground black pepper, to taste

- 1 tablespoons butter

Instructions

1. Take a bowl and whisk eggs with all the remaining ingredients in it.

2. Then take a skillet and heat butter.

3. Pour the ¼ of egg mixture into your skillet.

4. After that, cook for 2 minutes per side.

5. Repeat to use the entire batter.

6. Serve warm and enjoy!

Preparation Time: 5 minutes **Servings:** 2

Cooking Time: 20 minutes

Nutrition: Calories: 141 Fat: 11.5g Carbohydrates: 0.6g Protein: 8.9g Fiber: 0g Net Carbohydrates: 0.5g

SPRING SALAD

Ingredients:

- 2 ounce Mixed Green Vegetables

- 3 tablespoon roasted pine nuts

- 2 tablespoon 5 minutes 5 Keto Raspberry Vinaigrette

- 2 tablespoon Shaved Parmesan

- 2 slices bacon

- Salt, as required

- Pepper, as required

Instructions

1. Take a cooking pan and add bacon, cook the bacon until crispy.

2. Take a bowl and add the salad ingredients and mix well, add crumbled bacon into the salad.

3. Mix well.

4. Dress it with your favorite dressing.

5. Enjoy!

Preparation Time: 10-15 minutes **Servings:** 2

Cooking Time: 0 minutes

Nutrition: Calories: 209 Fat: 17g Net Carbohydrates: 10g Protein: 4g Fiber: 2g Carbohydrates: 12g

CHOCOLATE BERRY PROTEIN BARS

Ingredients:

- ½ cup almonds, sliced

- 1 cup chocolate protein powder

- ½ cup pecan pieces

- ½ cup fresh cherries, pitted

- ¼ cup fresh blueberries

- ¼ cup unsweetened coconut, shredded

- ½ cup almond butter

- ¼ cup of coconut oil

- ¼ cup almond meal

- 1 teaspoon vanilla

- 2 whole eggs

- ½ teaspoon salt

Instructions

1. Take a loaf pan and grease it.

2. Preheat your oven to 325 degrees Fahrenheit.

3. Take a bowl and add all of the listed ingredients except fruit.

4. Fold in berries and cherries into the batter.

5. Pour into the pan.

6. Bake for 10 minutes.

7. Let it cool for 10 minutes.

8. Cut into 12 bars and enjoy!

Preparation Time: 4 minutes **Servings:** 2

Cooking Time: 10 minutes

Nutrition: Calories: 235 Fat: 17g Net Carbohydrates: 6g Protein: 8g Fiber: 2g Carbohydrates: 8g

CAULIFLOWER RICE

Ingredients:

- 1 head cauliflower head, grated

- 1 tablespoon soy sauce

- 1 pinch salt

- 1 pinch black pepper

- 1 tablespoon garlic powder

- 1 tablespoon sesame oil

Instructions

1. Add cauliflower to a food processor and grate it.

2. Take a pan and add sesame oil, let it heat up over medium heat.

3. Add grated cauliflower and pour soy sauce.

4. Cook for 4-6 minutes.

5. Season and enjoy it!

Preparation Time: 5 minutes **Servings:** 2

Cooking Time: 6 minutes

Nutrition: Calories: 329 Fat: 28g Net Carbohydrates: 13g Protein: 10g Fiber: 2g Carbohydrates: 15g

CAULIFLOWER BERRY BREAKFAST BOWL

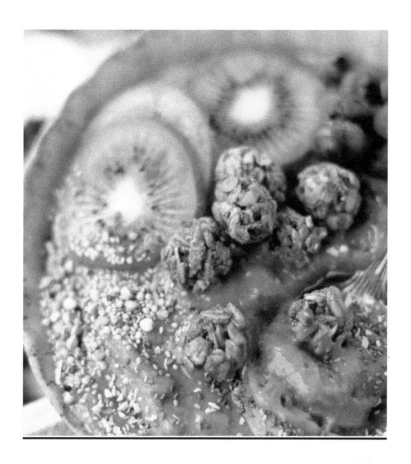

Ingredients:

- ½ cup cauliflower, frozen

- ¼ cup zucchini, frozen

- 1 cup fresh spinach

- ½ cup frozen raspberries

- 1 cup unsweetened almond milk

- 2 tbsp. almond butter

- 3 tbsp. chia seeds

- 1 tsp ground cinnamon

Instructions

- Add all ingredients to a blender. Place the frozen ingredients closest to the blades. Blend until smooth and creamy consistency is achieved and all the ingredients are well incorporated.

- Divide the mixture between serving bowls. Can be topped with fresh raspberries and serve.

Preparation Time: 15 minutes **Servings:** 6

Cooking Time: 0 minutes

Nutrition: Total fat: 8g Cholesterol: 0mg Sodium: 40mg Total carbohydrates: 13.8g Dietary fiber: 7.1g

Protein: 4.3g Calcium: 155mg Potassium: 220mg Iron: 3mg Vitamin D: 0mcg

NO - FUSS BREAKFAST CEREAL

Ingredients:

- 1 cup unsweetened coconut flakes

- ½ cup raw pumpkin seeds

- ½ cup sunflower seeds

- ¼ cup chia seeds

- 1 tbsp. toasted sesame seeds

- ¼ cup coconut oil

- 1 1/2 tsp vanilla extract

- A pinch of salt

- Coconut milk and fresh berries, like blackberries or blueberries for serving

Instructions

1. Preheat your oven to 300 degrees F.

2. Prepare a baking sheet by lining it with parchment paper.

3. In a large mixing bowl, add coconut flakes, pumpkin seeds, sunflower seeds, chia seeds, sesame seeds and salt. Mix well.

4. Add coconut oil and vanilla extract. Mix again.

5. Spread mixture onto prepared baking sheet in an even layer.

6. Bake for 20 minutes or until cereal golden brown. Stir halfway through.

7. Remove cereal from oven and allow cereal to cool to preference. Serve with coconut milk and berries

Preparation Time: 15 minutes **Servings:** 8

Cooking Time: 20 minutes

Nutrition: Total fat: 18.7g Cholesterol: 0mg Sodium: 23mg Total carbohydrates: 8g Dietary fiber: 4.4g

Protein: 4.7g Calcium: 62mg Potassium: 124mg Iron: 2mg Vitamin D: 0mcg

EASY BREAKFAST BAGELS

Ingredients:

- 1 cup ground flax seed

- 1 cup tahini

- ½ cup psyllium husks

- 2 cup water 2 tsp baking powder

- A pinch of salt

Instructions

1. Preheat your oven to 375 degrees F.

2. Prepare a baking sheet by lining it with parchment paper.

3. Add flax seeds, psyllium husk, baking powder and salt to a bowl. Whisk to combine.

4. In a small bowl, whisk together water and tahini. Pour into dry ingredients and fold in. Knead to form the dough.

Create 12 circles about 4" in diameter, and 1/4" **Instructions**

5. thick.

6. Place circles on prepared baking sheet, spaced equally apart. Cut a small circle from the middle of each circle.

7. Bake for around 40 minutes or until golden brown.

8. Remove from oven and allow to cool.

9. Cut in half and top as desired. Serve.

Preparation Time: 20 minutes **Servings:** 12

Cooking Time: 40 minutes

Nutrition: Total fat: 13.7g Cholesterol: 0mg Sodium: 95mg Total carbohydrates: 29.8g Dietary fiber: 23.2g Protein: 5.1g Calcium: 125mg Potassium: 247mg Iron: 5mg Vitamin D: 0mcg

CRANBERRY BREAKFAST BARS

Ingredients:

- 1/3 cup dried cranberries

- 1 cup pecans

- 1 cup water

- ¼ cup coconut butter, softened

- 2 tbsp. granulated erythritol

- 1 tbsp. ground flax seed

- 2 tsp allspice blend

- 1 ½ tsp baking powder

- 1 tsp vanilla extract

Instructions

1. Preheat your oven to 350 degrees F.

2. Prepare an 8x8 brownie pan by lining it with parchment paper.

3. Add all ingredients to a blender and blend until slightly lumpy consistency is achieved.

4. Pour mixture into prepared brownie pan. Use a spatula to smooth the top.

5. Bake for 45 minutes or until a toothpick comes out clean when inserted into the center.

6. Remove the pan from the oven and allow to cool completely before removing and slicing into individual bars. If you do not allow the bars to cool completely then they will fall apart. Serve

Preparation Time: 10 minutes **Servings:** 10

Cooking Time: 45 minutes

Nutrition: Total fat: 15.7g Cholesterol: 0mg Sodium: 5mg Total carbohydrates: 6.3g Dietary fiber: 3.4g Protein: 2.3g Calcium: 49mg Potassium: 151mg Iron: 1mg Vitamin D: 0mcg

PUMPKIN SPICE PANCAKES

Ingredients:

- ¼ cup pumpkin puree

- 1/3 cup almond milk

- 1/3 cup coconut flour

- 1/3 cup water

- 1/3 cup almond flour

- ¼ tsp baking soda

- 1 tbsp. vanilla protein powder

- 1/8 tsp ground cinnamon

- 1/8 tsp ground ginger

- 1 tsp stevia powder

Instructions

1. Add coconut flour, almond flours, baking soda, cinnamon, ginger, stevia and protein powder to a mixing bowl. Mix well.

2. Add almond milk, water and pumpkin puree to a blender and blend to a smooth consistency. Pour into dry ingredients and combine until no lumps are visible.

3. Grease a nonstick skillet and place on medium heat. Add 1/4 cup of batter to heated skillet at a time. Cook for 1 minute or until the bottom edges turn golden brown. Flip and cook for 1 more minute. Repeat until all batter is used up.

4. Remove, plate and serve with toppings such as fresh berries or berry jam.

Preparation Time: 23 minutes **Servings:** 6

Cooking Time: 2 minutes

Nutrition: Total fat: 6.1g Cholesterol: 0mg Sodium: 3mg Total carbohydrates: 5.9g Dietary fiber: 3.5g

Protein: 1.3g Calcium: 27mg Potassium: 222mg Iron: 1mg Vitamin D: 0mcg

LEMON PANCAKES

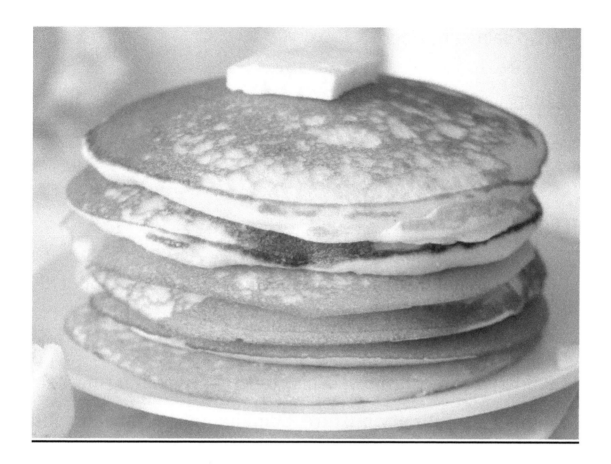

Ingredients:

- ½ tsp vanilla extract

- 1 tbsp. lemon juice

- 2 tbsp. coconut butter, melted

- 1 tbsp. granulated erythritol

- 5 tbsp. almond milk

- ¼ cup coconut flour

- ½ tsp baking powder

- 1 tbsp. psyllium husk

- A pinch of salt

Instructions

1. In a medium mixing bowl, whisk together coconut flour, baking powder, salt and psyllium.

2. In a large mixing bowl, whisk together remaining ingredients then stir into dry mixture. Combine thoroughly and ensure that there are no lumps.

3. Allow the mixture to sit for 5 minutes or until a stiff dough forms. You should be able to mold this dough with your hands. If not, stir in additional coconut flour.

4. Divide the dough into 5 equal portions to form 5 balls.

5. Heat a nonstick skillet over medium heat. Grease with coconut oil.

6. Flatten dough and add to pan. Cook for 5 minutes on each side or until golden brown and cooked through.

7. Allow to cool for a few minutes and serve.

Preparation Time: 55 minutes **Servings:** 6

Cooking Time: 5 minutes

Nutrition: Total fat: 18.5g Cholesterol: 0mg Sodium: 52mg Total carbohydrates: 16.6g Dietary fiber: 11.2g Protein: 2.7g Calcium: 29mg Potassium: 80mg Iron: 1mg Vitamin D: 0mcg

KETO VEGAN VANILLA FRENCH TOAST

Ingredients:

- 5 slices fresh coconut bread (or any other keto vegan friendly sandwich bread)

- ¼ tsp ground cinnamon

- ¼ cup vanilla protein powder

- ½ cup almond milk

- A pinch of ground nutmeg

Instructions

1. Whisk together almond milk, protein powder, nutmeg and cinnamon in a shallow but wide dish that the bread can fit into. Ensure that there are no lumps in the mix.

2. Heat a nonstick skillet over medium heat and grease with coconut oil.

3. Soak each piece of bread in the vanilla protein powder mixture for 5 seconds on each side.

4. Place the soaked pieces of bread in the skillet and cook for 5 minutes so that the bottom turns golden brown. Flip and cook for another 5 minutes or until the other side is golden brown.

5. Plate and serve

Preparation Time: 10 minutes **Servings:** 5

Cooking Time: 10 minutes

Nutrition: Total fat: 8.3g Cholesterol: 0mg Sodium: 11mg Total carbohydrates: 23.5g Dietary fiber: 2.6g Protein: 3.9g Calcium: 12mg Potassium: 166mg Iron: 1mg Vitamin D: 0mcg

ALMOND SMOOTHIE

Ingredients:

- ¾ cup almonds, chopped

- ½ cup heavy whipping cream

- 2 teaspoons butter, melted

- ¼ teaspoon organic vanilla extract

- 7–8 drops liquid stevia

- 1 cup unsweetened almond milk

- ¼ cup ice cubes

Instructions

- In a blender, put all the listed Ingredients: and pulse until creamy.

- Pour the smoothie into two glasses and serve immediately.

Preparation Time: 10 minutes **Servings:** 2

Cooking Time: 10 minutes

Nutrition: Calories 365 Net Carbs 4.5 g Total Fat 34.55 g Saturated Fat 10.8 g Cholesterol 51 mg Sodium 129 mg Total Carbs 9.5 g Fiber 5 g Sugar 1.6 g Protein 8.7 g

MOCHA SMOOTHIE

Ingredients:

- 2 teaspoons instant espresso powder

- 2-3 tablespoons granulated erythritol

- 2 teaspoons cacao powder

- ½ cup plain Greek yogurt

- 1 cup unsweetened almond milk

- 1 cup ice cubes

Instructions

1. In a blender, put all the listed **Ingredients:** and pulse until creamy.

2. Pour the smoothie into two glasses and serve immediately.

Preparation Time: 10 minutes **Servings:** 2

Cooking Time: 10 minutes

Nutrition: Calories 70 Net Carbs 5.5 g Total Fat 2.8 g Saturated Fat 1 g Cholesterol 4 mg Sodium 133 mg Total Carbs 6.5 g Fiber 1 g Sugar 4.3 g Protein 4.4 g

STRAWBERRY SMOOTHIE

Ingredients:

- 4 ounces frozen strawberries

- 2 teaspoons granulated erythritol

- ½ teaspoon organic vanilla extract

- 1/3 cup heavy whipping cream

- 1¼ cups unsweetened almond milk

- ½ cup ice cubes

Instructions

1. In a blender, put all the listed Ingredients: and pulse until creamy.

2. Pour the smoothie into two glasses and serve immediately.

Preparation Time: 10 minutes **Servings:** 2

Cooking Time: 10 minutes

Nutrition: Calories 115 Net Carbs 4.5 g Total Fat 9.8 g Saturated Fat 4.8 g Cholesterol 27 mg Sodium 121 mg Total Carbs 6.3 g Fiber 1.8 g Sugar 2.9 g Protein 1.4 g

RASPBERRY SMOOTHIE

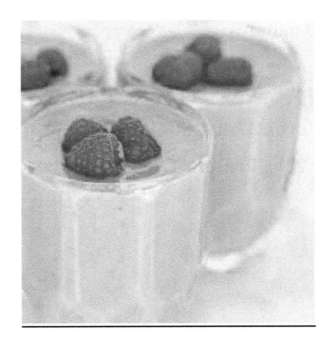

Ingredients:

- ¾ cup fresh raspberries

- 3 tablespoons heavy whipping cream

- 1/3 ounce cream cheese

- 1 cup unsweetened almond milk

- ½ cup ice, crushed

Instructions

1. In a blender, put all the listed Ingredients: and pulse until creamy.

2. Pour the smoothie into two glasses and serve immediately.

Preparation Time: 10 minutes **Servings:** 2

Cooking Time: 10 minutes

Nutrition: Calories 138 Net Carbs 3.8 g Total Fat 12 g Saturated Fat 6.4 g Cholesterol 36 mg Sodium 115 mg Total Carbs 7.3 g Fiber 3.5 g Sugar 2.1 g Protein 1.9 g

PUMPKIN SMOOTHIE

Ingredients:

- ½ cup homemade pumpkin puree

- 4 ounces cream cheese, softened

- ¼ cup heavy cream

- ½ teaspoon pumpkin pie spice

- ¼ teaspoon ground cinnamon

- 8 drops liquid stevia

- 1 teaspoon organic vanilla extract

- 1 cup unsweetened almond milk

- ¼ cup ice cubes

Instructions

1. In a blender, put all the listed Ingredients: and pulse until creamy.

2. Pour the smoothie into two glasses and serve immediately.

Preparation Time: 10 minutes **Servings:** 2

Cooking Time: 10 minutes

Nutrition: Calories 296 Net Carbs 5.4 g Total Fat 27.1 g Saturated Fat 16.1g Cholesterol 83 mg Sodium 266 mg Total Carbs 8 g Fiber 2.6 g Sugar 2.4 g Protein 5.6 g

SPINACH & AVOCADO SMOOTHIE

Ingredients:

- ½ large avocado, peeled, pitted, and roughly chopped

- 2 cups fresh spinach

- 1 tablespoon MCT oil

- 1 teaspoon organic vanilla extract

- 6–8 drops liquid stevia

- 1½ cups unsweetened almond milk

- ½ cup ice cubes

Instructions

1. In a blender, put all the listed **Ingredients:** and pulse until creamy.

2. Pour the smoothie into two glasses and serve immediately.

Preparation Time: 10 minutes **Servings:** 2

Cooking Time: 10 minutes

Nutrition: Calories 180 Net Carbs 0 g Total Fat 18 g Saturated Fat 9 g Cholesterol 0 mg Sodium 161 mg Total Carbs 6.5 g Fiber 4.3 g Sugar 0.6 g Protein 2.4 g

MATCHA SMOOTHIE

Ingredients:

- 2 tablespoons chia seeds

- 2 teaspoons matcha green tea powder

- ½ teaspoon fresh lemon juice

- ½ teaspoon xanthan gum

- 10 drops liquid stevia

- 4 tablespoons plain Greek yogurt

- 1½ cups unsweetened almond milk

- ¼ cup ice cubes

Instructions

- In a blender, put all the listed **Ingredients:** and pulse until creamy.

- Pour the smoothie into two glasses and serve immediately.

Preparation Time: 10 minutes **Servings:** 2

Cooking Time: 10 minutes

Nutrition: Calories 85 Net Carbs 3.5 g Total Fat 5.5 g Saturated Fat 0.8 g Cholesterol 2 mg Sodium 174 mg Total Carbs 7.6 g Fiber 4.1 g Sugar 2.2 g Protein 4 g

Creamy Spinach Smoothie

Ingredients:

- 2 cups fresh baby spinach

- 1 tablespoon almond butter

- 1 tablespoon chia seeds

- 1/8 teaspoon ground cinnamon

- Pinch of ground cloves

- ½ cup heavy cream

- 1 cup unsweetened almond milk

- ½ cup ice cubes

Instructions

1. In a blender, put all the listed **Ingredients:** and pulse until creamy.

2. Pour the smoothie into two glasses and serve immediately.

Preparation Time: 10 minutes **Servings:** 2

Cooking Time: 10 minutes

Nutrition: Calories 195 Net Carbs 2.8 g Total Fat 18.8 g Saturated Fat 7.5 g Cholesterol 41 mg Sodium 126 mg Total Carbs 6.1 g Fiber 3.3 g Sugar 0.5 g Protein 4.5 g

CONCLUSIONE

Here we are at the end of this wonderful journey, full of flavor and energy. Did you enjoy the recipes?

Did you have breakfast with the whole family?

I recommend that you always consult with a nutritionist or medical professional before starting any diet, and practice making these delicious recipes to your very best.

Hugs to you and thank you.

CPSIA information can be obtained
at www.ICGtesting.com
Printed in the USA
LVHW060344280421
685801LV00014B/960